Learn to Let Go

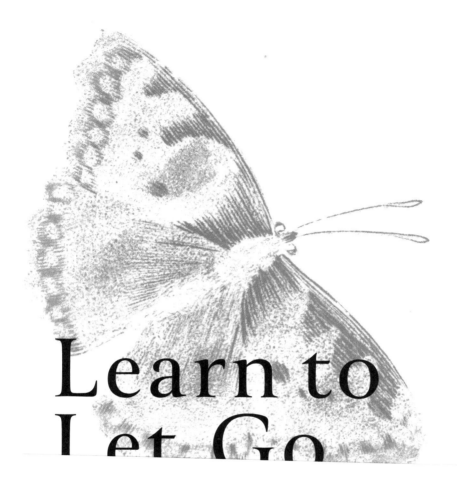

Learn to
Let Go

This journal belongs to

_____

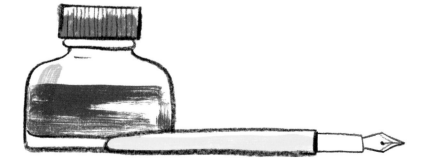

For the Explorer in all of us.

First published in Great Britain in 2023 by Aster,
an imprint of Octopus Publishing Group Ltd,
Carmelite House, 50 Victoria Embankment,
London EC4Y 0DZ
www.octopusbooks.co.uk

An Hachette UK Company
www.hachette.co.uk

Distributed in the US by Hachette Book Group,
1290 Avenue of the Americas, 4th and 5th Floors
New York, NY 10104

Distributed in Canada by Canadian Manda Group,
664 Annette St, Toronto, Ontario, Canada M6S 2C8

ISBN 978-1-78325-543-6

A CIP catalogue record for this book is available from the British Library.

Printed and bound in China.

1 3 5 7 9 10 8 6 4 2

Note: If the exercises included in this book bring up memories that feel too painful to deal with
by yourself, please do seek professional help, either through your GP, who can refer you
to professional counselling services, or through a professional therapist.

Commissioner: Nicola Crane
Senior Editor: Leanne Bryan
Art Director: Yasia Williams
Copyeditor: Monica Hope
Designer: Siaron Hughes
Illustrator: Ella McLean
Assistant Production Manager: Allison Gonsalves

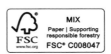

Contents

Introduction

What do you want to change in your life? Maybe you want better health, a relationship, happier relationships, a better job or more money. Or maybe you want less of something, like stress or frustration, or fewer problems with your boss. Maybe you've been trying to change your life for years, but it still hasn't happened – which has left you feeling stuck.

In *The Power of Letting Go*, I showed you how to live life on another level, so you could see yourself and the world around you in a completely different way, and let go of years of conditioning. This conditioning had led you to believe that the only way to make things happen is to think hard, take lots of action and keep going through thick and thin. *Learn to Let Go* will now give you the steps to make things happen much more easily, with a lot less stress.

You don't need to control everything that's happening. You don't need to push, struggle, fight or force things or try to manipulate people in order to make things the way you want them to be. That's exhausting and unnecessary. If you let go in the way I described in *The Power of Letting Go*, and follow the exercises in this journal, you'll experience what's often called 'flow'. You'll find yourself working in sync with the world instead of fighting against it. When you let go, your intuition will become much stronger. While it's OK to have a plan, it's also essential to tune in to what's actually happening and work with it instead of against it. You'll be much more successful at whatever you choose to do.

You can let go in three stages. For most of us, letting go is a gradual process. Right now, you may not even be aware of what's holding you back. The three stages are:

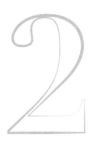

Let go of thoughts, including judgements, labels, expectations and stories. For example, you realize that your mind keeps creating problems by chattering on about something that has no relevance to what's happening now. You learn to witness – or observe – the thoughts and let them go. Now you can get on with life.

Let go of pain, which is provoked by a constant stream of negative thoughts. For example, there may be a painful memory that makes it very hard for you to live life to the full. You re-live the experience and allow yourself to feel the pain, suffering, discomfort or agitation. It gradually dies down, and is highly likely to disappear. Your mind is clearer and you feel much better.

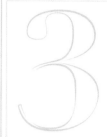

Surrender and tune in to something far more intelligent than your brain. Now that you've let go of the past and the future, you fall into the present. You follow your intuition and naturally take the right action at the right time. Everything happens more easily.

Good things happen when you let go. You feel more relaxed and forget to worry, you understand intuitively what's going on around you, things fall into place, you take the right action at the right time, your health improves, relationships are easy, you allow other people to be as they are, and you laugh more. Once you learn to let go, your desires can be fulfilled easily and without stress.

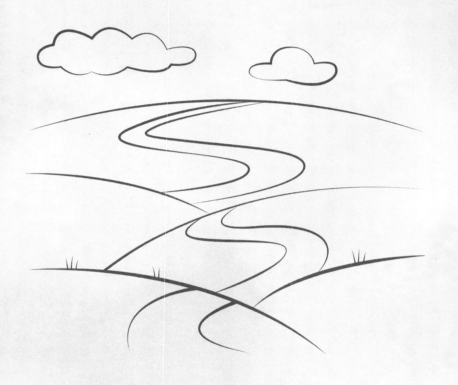

Make your own discoveries while you use this journal. Science is widely misunderstood. Some people 'believe in science' the way others 'believe in religion'. But science isn't a belief system, it's a method of enquiry. The scientific method is ultimately about letting go – in a systematic fashion – of all the flawed theories and explanations that our minds make up.

We can never prove something to be true. We can only discover what's false, thereby getting closer to the truth. My recommendation is that you simply try the exercises in this book and see what happens. Just give it a go.

Some of the exercises require a few minutes of dedicated time. You can practise the others in the middle of whatever else you're doing. They've worked for large numbers of people, but not every exercise works for everyone. Try each one for yourself as you read this journal. In some cases you may notice a difference – or learn something – right away. In other cases, nothing may happen, at least initially, so I suggest you move on and come back to it later. An exercise that does nothing for you the first time you try it may prove very useful later on.

If you do the exercises thoroughly, you'll start noticing benefits in every area of your life.

The good news is that you can let go all the time. You don't have to be on top of a mountain, in a yoga pose or deep in meditation to let go. You can let go all day long, right where you are, while doing whatever you're doing. That's what this journal will show you, step by step. Once you settle into it, you'll wonder why you ever tried living any other way. When we let go completely we're more fulfilled than ever before – with little or no stress.

Let's get started.

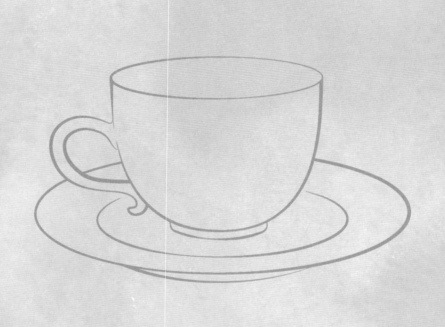

Be Present and
Enjoy Each Moment

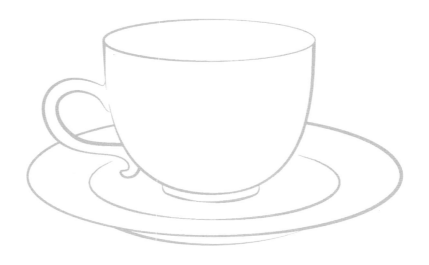

Being present is essential preparation for the three key steps in this journal, which are to:

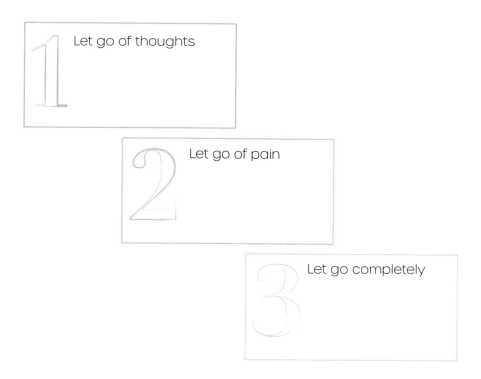

1 Let go of thoughts

2 Let go of pain

3 Let go completely

You're physically present all the time – it's only your attention that wanders. Left to its own devices, our attention runs around, out of control. Being present simply means that we bring our attention back to the present moment. It sounds simple, but putting it into practice requires specific techniques.

All the techniques described in this chapter will help you to be present. This allows life to unfold naturally, including the things you want to happen.

Start meditating

Lots of people try meditation and quickly give up. Some say they tried without any instructions, but most just say they found it impossible to control their minds.

Just so you know what you're up against, try this exercise.

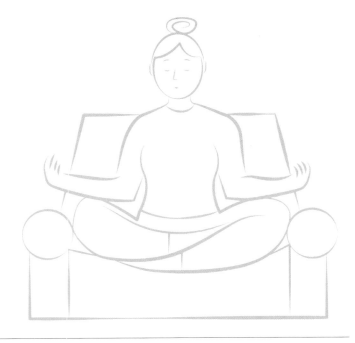

Exercise

Sit in a quiet place where you won't be disturbed. Switch off your phone. Close your eyes. For the next five minutes, stop thinking.

•••

How did you get on? You may have found it impossible to stop thinking for more than a few seconds. After a while, a thought appears, then another, then another. Pretty soon you're thinking about the future or the past, or about what may be happening somewhere else right now.

Jot down some bullet points in the space below, describing the thoughts that popped into your head:

_____

_____

_____

_____

_____

_____

_____

_____

_____

_____

_____

_____

_____

_____

The secret to meditation

A lot of people think meditation is about emptying the mind, but most of us find that impossible – at least initially. So, what's the answer?

The secret of meditation is to give the mind something to do. This exercise is an easy way to get started.

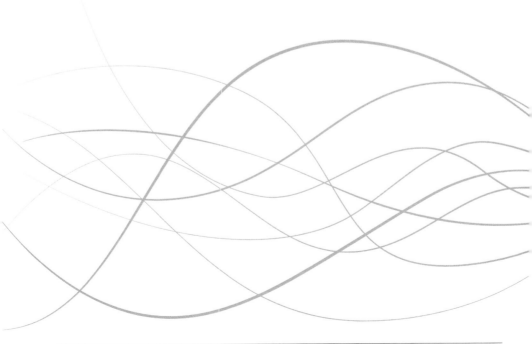

Exercise

- Sit in a quiet place where you won't be disturbed. Switch off your phone and take off your watch. Close your eyes.

- Now turn your attention inwards. Place your attention on your breath as it flows in and out.

- Every time your attention wanders, bring it gently back to the breath. There's no need to judge yourself – it's all part of the process. Just relax and bring your attention back to the breath.

- Carry on doing this for several minutes.

• • •

Now open your eyes. What do you notice? How do you feel? Do you notice any difference in the sounds, colours or shapes around you? Use the space below to write down what you've observed:

_____

_____

_____

_____

_____

_____

_____

_____

_____

_____

_____

Connect with your senses

Let's extend this meditation exercise from your breath to your five senses. The following exercise is from the School of Philosophy and Economic Science; according to tradition, it goes back thousands of years. It's fine to glance at your watch occasionally while you're meditating. Then you can bring your attention back to the breath. Often when people meditate in groups, there's someone who keeps track of time, ringing a bell at the beginning and the end. Doing this exercise in the morning will help your day get off to a great start.

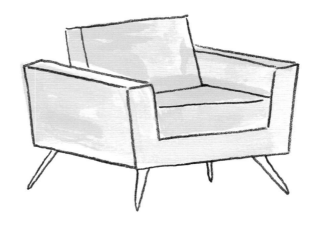

Exercise

- Find a quiet place where you won't be disturbed.

- Sit upright on a chair, completely relaxed. Place your hands on your thighs and your feet flat on the floor. Close your eyes.

- Allow your body to relax. Let go of any tension.
Let go of any concerns or preoccupations.

- Place your attention on the breath as it flows in and out. Every time your attention wanders, bring it gently back to your breath.

- Now feel the air on your face. Be aware of this for a while.

- Now feel the weight of your body on the chair.
Be aware of this for a while.

- Every time your attention wanders, bring it gently back to the breath.

- Now feel the touch of your feet on the ground.
Be aware of this for a while.

- Listen as far as possible into the distance, beyond the sounds nearby.
Be aware of this for a while.

- Let go of any mental comments or judgements about the sounds.

- Now bring your attention back to the breath as it flows in and out.

- Every time your attention wanders, bring it gently back
to your breath.

Observe the thoughts as they come and go

While you were doing the last two exercises, you may have noticed now and then that there weren't any thoughts. Maybe it only lasted for a second or two. As soon as you realize *I've stopped thinking*, that's another thought. But that gap between thoughts was pure consciousness.

Many of us believe we *are* our thoughts – and behave accordingly. We have a happy thought, so we feel happy. We have a sad thought, so we feel sad. In other words, *we identify* with our thoughts.

The solution is to stand back from your thoughts and observe them as they come and go. Being present will help you. If you can observe something, it isn't you. You're the observer, not the thought or feeling (such as discomfort, frustration or annoyance).

Exercise

- Close your eyes if it's safe to do so. Otherwise, place your attention on an object in front of you.

- Now feel the breath moving slowly in and out of your body. Feel the weight of your body on the chair, and then the touch of your feet on the floor. Feel the texture of whatever your hands are touching. Every time your attention wanders, bring it gently back to one of your senses. If you feel angry or frustrated, notice that feeling and then bring your attention back to your senses.

- Don't deny or repress any thoughts or feelings that may come up. All you're doing is noticing them, and then bringing your attention back to your senses.

•••

Now try this:

- Notice each thought as it appears. Don't try to do anything about it. Don't judge it, resist it or push it away. Just witness it, observe it.

- In a while the thought will disappear, and another thought will come. Just let them come and go.

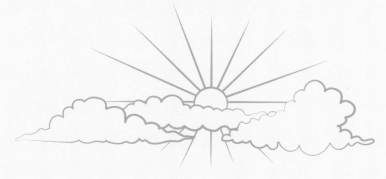

Practise being present

'When an inner situation is not made consciuos, it happens outside, as fate'

– Carl Jung, *Aion*

Being present will help you avoid making decisions that you later regret. The more present you are, the easier it'll be to observe thoughts and then decide whether you're going to act on them. You'll become more and more aware of what's going on around you – and in your mind. You're much less likely to be a victim of 'fate'.

Being present in this way can help you see things clearly before you decide to act. It reduces stress. It also helps us let go of fear, stay safe, keep cool and enjoy harmonious relationships.

Exercise

Think of a situation in which you found someone's mood or behaviour stressful or you felt under pressure – during a job interview, a sporting competition or a public-speaking event, for example. Write about it in the space below:

_____

_____

_____

_____

_____

_____

_____

_____

_____

_____

_____

_____

Now you have a choice: you can either allow your mind to run wild in these moments, or you can be present.

If you keep your attention on your breath, your senses and your surroundings, you'll remain in the present moment. You won't become nearly as stressed.

Watch the thoughts and emotions come and go

Sometimes thoughts and emotions come thick and fast, particularly if someone has criticized you or tried to harm you. When this happens, it's best to stand back from it all. Try the following exercise:

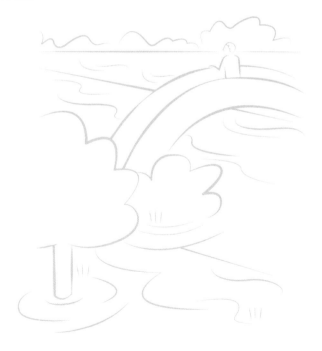

Exercise

• Imagine that it's raining hard and you're standing on a bridge over a river that is close to bursting its banks. The swirling water is your mind in chaos. The river is becoming more and more dangerous, carrying all kinds of debris with it. There are branches from dead trees, wooden planks and car tyres caught in the swell.

• The debris is your thoughts and emotions. There may be unpleasant memories of what someone said about you, maybe a few negative thoughts you've had about yourself and about what might go wrong now. Along with the thoughts comes a stream of negative emotions such as anger, sadness, regret and the feeling you're not good enough. They all come sweeping down the river.

• There's no need for you to reach down and grab hold of them. If you do so, you may be dragged along and swept away. All you have to do is be present. Feel the weight of your feet on the bridge. Feel the sensations in your body and the breath flowing in and out. Imagine the thoughts and emotions rushing by beneath you. Imagine you're resting your hands on the wall of the bridge, and looking down into the water. Feel the stone wall beneath your hands.

• Whenever you get distracted, bring your attention back to your breath. Breathe slowly and deeply. Place your attention within your body. Observe the thoughts and emotions – allow them to come and go.

Practise mindfulness during the day

Being present, while calmly acknowledging your thoughts, emotions and bodily sensations, is often described as 'mindfulness'. If you practise mindfulness a couple of times a day – sitting on your own in a quiet place – it will gradually spill over into your whole life.

Each activity is an opportunity to keep your attention in the here and now. You could be washing the dishes or walking down the street.

Try the following exercise:

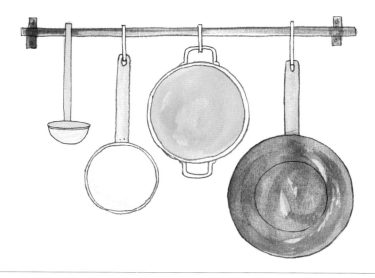

Exercise

• Stand up and walk around slowly. Feel your feet pressing into the ground and the breath flowing in and out of your body.

• Every now and then you may notice that your attention has wandered. Suddenly you're immersed in thoughts about the past or the future, or what might be happening somewhere else right now. As soon as you notice this, bring your attention back to the present using one of your senses. One way is to press your thumbnails into your forefingers. A bit of discomfort can be useful – it gets our attention.

Ideas and solutions come from not thinking

Maybe you've experienced something like this:

- You work on a problem until you get stuck and can't go any further.

- You do something physical such as walking, swimming or playing sport.

- The solution comes to you in a flash, either during the activity or shortly afterwards when you look at the problem again.

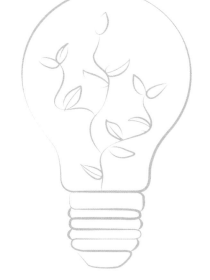

Exercise

When has a solution appeared after you stopped thinking and let go?
Write it down to remind yourself:

The 'I am' mantra

Practices such as mindfulness and yoga help us to think a lot less in our daily lives and just *be*. We begin to return to our original state. As babies we simply are – we radiate love. As we grow up, we start to identify with all kinds of things. We start to believe that we are our bodies, which can make us obsessed with each change that occurs and afraid of death. Many of us believe that we are the mind – the endless mental chatter that demands a response, with the compulsion to analyse everyone and everything.

Think about it for a moment. You were none of these things when you were born. You'll let go of all of them when you die. So what happens in between? The answer is that you're pure consciousness, which you may experience for a few seconds if you wake up gently without an alarm. Then – within a few seconds – your mind will start chattering about your concerns, responsibilities, tea, coffee, breakfast and so on.

If you meditate correctly, you may experience pure consciousness. There's no identity, no thoughts or beliefs, no story about what's happened, is happening or will happen. There's just consciousness.

Exercise

- For this exercise, either go for a walk or sit somewhere quiet. While you're walking around, or sitting somewhere, keep thinking one thought: 'I am.'

- If any other thoughts occur to you – which they almost certainly will – go back to this thought. If you notice that you've started to identify, let go. Return to the thought, 'I am.'

Keep thinking it over and over again, like a mantra. (It *is* a mantra.)

• • •

You can use this mantra anywhere, at any time. Here are two examples:

- If you're engaged in some vigorous activity such as running, try thinking, 'I am,' over and over again. You may notice the 'I am' coinciding with the in- and out-breaths, while your body carries on doing what it needs to do.

- If your mind goes into overdrive, speculating about what might happen or could happen, focus simply on 'I am'. If you keep your mind focused on 'I am', you may find that the torrent of thoughts dies down.

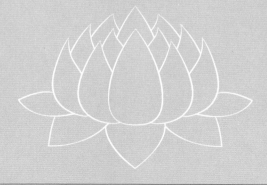

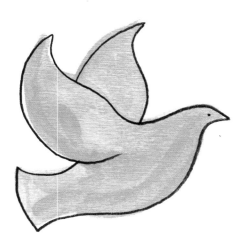

Let Go of the Thoughts That Keep You Stuck

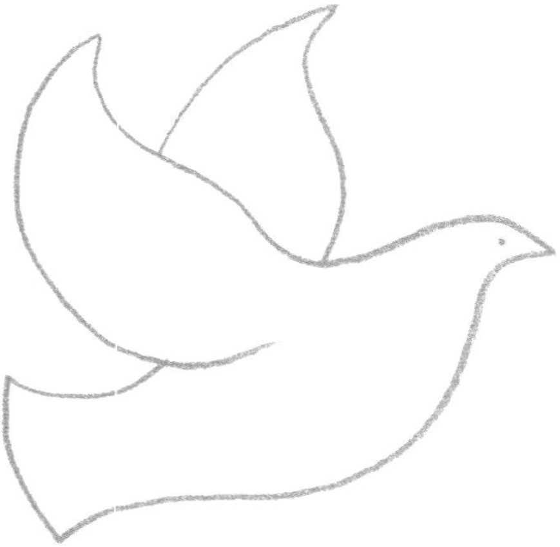

Once you've learned to be present and observe your thoughts, you can start letting go of them.

You may be wondering why this is a good idea. The answer is that repetitive thoughts keep you stuck and prevent things from happening in your life. Here are some examples:

- Thoughts about the past

- Thoughts about the future, including worries and *if onlys*

- Stories

- Labels

- Judgements

- Expectations

- Comparisons

- Opinions

- Conclusions

- Conspiracy theories.

These thoughts prevent us from seeing and hearing what's going on, and from absorbing information and exploring new opportunities. They block our intuition and stop useful ideas from coming to us. When we let go of repetitive thoughts, we allow things to happen in new and exciting ways.

Let go of the past

Our thoughts and feelings about the past get in the way of what's happening now. Letting go of them creates space for new things to happen.

Constantly connecting the present with the past prevents us from experiencing life as it unfolds. It can also feel dull and heavy. It's usually easier to observe this in other people than in ourselves. You've probably met someone who keeps reacting to events in the present by talking about the past. You may also have noticed the same tendency in yourself – the past gets in the way of the present. (It's particularly hard to get to know a potential partner if you keep comparing them with your ex.)

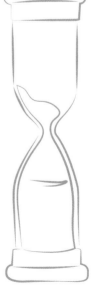

Exercise

Next time you're listening to someone, you may notice that your mind
has drawn a comparison with the past.

Now you have a choice:

• You could choose to talk about the past. Maybe you can predict which
way the conversation will go if you do that.

• You could say nothing about the past. In fact, you could say nothing at
all, and then see what happens next. Give it a try. What happens now?

• • •

• This exercise takes practice. Someone may say something and then
you find yourself talking at length about the past. When this happens,
you can simply ask a question and get them talking again. Then listen
and see what happens.

If there's a pause in the conversation, *let it be*. Something will happen.
It needn't be you talking about the past again.

Let go of the future

'True happiness is to enjoy the present, without anxious dependence on the future'

– Lucius Annaeus Seneca

The future isn't a problem. It's only your ego that worries about the future. If you identify with your body or mind then you'll automatically have anxious thoughts about what will happen, what could happen and so on. We've been conditioned to see life as a fight for survival. This journal will help you let go of the ego and experience yourself as consciousness.

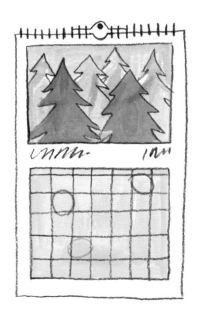

Exercise

Be clear about what you want to happen. For example, it could be moving
to a new house or finding a new job or business opportunity.

• Write it down here, and/or assemble some related images and stick
them below. Keep your focus on what you *do* want to happen, not what
you *don't* want to happen.

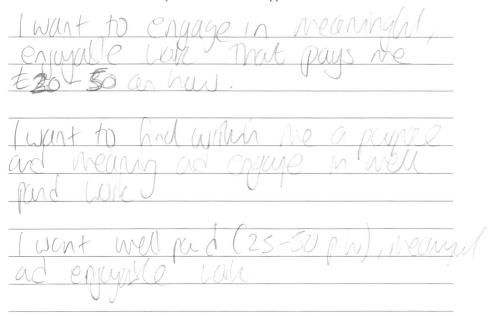

I want to engage in meaningful,
enjoyable work that pays me
£20 - 50 an hour.

I want to find within me a purpose
and meaning and engage in well
paid work

I want well paid (25-50 p.h), meaningful
and enjoyable work

Now bring your attention back to the present moment, using the
exercises described earlier in this journal. Let go of all your concerns
while you focus on your breath and your senses. Do this every time
you feel anxious. The more you remain present, the more clearly your
intuition will tell you what to do.

Let go of your stories

The best way to live is to experience each moment and then let it go. However, most of us don't do that. We label our experiences and assemble them to create stories – about ourselves, other people and the world around us.

We tell these stories to ourselves and to others – and we live by them. Some of our stories are based on painful events in the past but they shape the present and our future, causing lots more pain. There's no need to keep talking about them or allow them to take over our lives. Things become a lot more complicated once we start assembling stories about our *thoughts* and *feelings*. For example, 'I keep having problems with...', 'I don't want to show off', 'I'm unlucky in love', 'I'm a victim of...', 'I'm not good enough'.

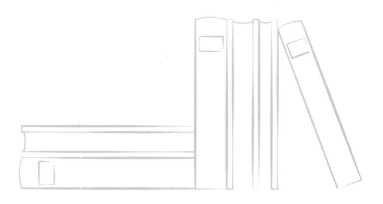

Exercise

Select one of the negative stories you tell about yourself and write down
the answers to the following questions:

What's the story you tell about yourself?

That something so bad happened when I was a
child -10 or 11- that 'ruined me' and the
effect has been that I have not prospered in
my career or had enough confidence to go for
something. May if only cut me off from
('many' myself (my 'latest story)

What are the beliefs underlying your story?

That the past has the power to control me
That I am damaged or different or
special in some way
That I am not good enough worthy
to do new that I don't have relevant skills
or experience

What short-term pleasure or comfort do you get from holding
on to each belief?

I don't have to take responsibility. Seek
sympathy + attention. Pleasure of self-pity.'
Ego feels special + different
Stay in the comfort zone I've always
been in -

What's the pay-off from telling this story?

Don't have to take responsibility
[obany others]. Stay in familiar
territory. Don't have to feel in any
[unusual] way.

What's this story costing you?

My life. [Sense] of achievement
and accomplishment. Makes me
spend my days bored + frustrated.
Lack of connection with others.
Not feeling part of the world.
[Isolation].

What will be the benefit to you from letting go of this story now?

Feel freer, connect — a desire
to connect to my real self. Improve
my relationships. [Lighter]. Energy
to start day differently. Opportunity
[what] meaning + purpose. A
more peaceful [mind].

Select another of your negative stories and carry out the same process.

What's the story you tell about yourself?

My life was ruined by my husbands affair. I've never gotten over the betrayal + subsequent divorce. That this impacted me and as a result could never build another relationship.

What are the beliefs underlying your story?

That [illegible] my married would have been better
That I was a victim
That we are here were breif
That my husband behaved selfishly

What short-term pleasure or comfort do you get from holding
on to each belief?

Live life as a victim + people can feel sorry for me and [illegible] term sympathy as a victim

Exercise (continued)

What's the pay-off from telling this story?

I protect myself from future pain
in an effort to feel safe.

What's this story costing you?

A new relationship.
Better relationships?
Peace + happiness
Contentment

What will be the benefit to you from letting go of this story now?

Peace + acceptance
Letting go of sadness

Let go of your stories about other people

You may also discover that you have stories about others. For example, 'People are so rude', 'Everyone's out for themselves', 'They're all a bunch of show-offs', 'All politicians are liars'.

Exercise

Write down your stories about other people and repeat the exercise:

What's the story you tell about others?

_____

_____

_____

_____

What are the beliefs underlying this story?

_____

_____

_____

_____

What short-term pleasure do you get from holding on to each belief?

_____

_____

_____

_____

_____

What's the pay-off from telling this story?

_____

_____

_____

_____

_____

_____

What's this story costing you?

_____

_____

_____

_____

_____

_____

What will be the benefit to you from letting go of this story now?

_____

_____

_____

_____

_____

_____

_____

Interrupt your stories

Positive stories can be just as limiting – for example, 'I'm a winner', 'I'm an achiever', 'I'm a good father', 'I'm intelligent'. This may be hard to grasp at first, particularly if you grew up in a Western culture. We've been heavily conditioned to see ourselves as separate, individual body/minds, trying to get what we want in competition with lots of other body/minds.

The reality is that we aren't the body or the mind, since we can observe our bodies and the ever-changing thoughts that we call the mind. We're the observer standing on the bridge. We're consciousness, which never changes. Everything else comes and goes. Letting go of your identity allows you to live from consciousness, which is infinitely powerful. Take the leap and experience it for yourself.

Exercise

Every time you notice that your mind is telling one of its stories, bring your attention back to the present. Choose an object and focus your attention on it. It could be a building, a tree, a cup or one of your fingernails. Look at it really carefully – study it.

You may notice that the story has stopped. If your mind wanders, the story may start up again. All you have to do is focus your attention on another object and study it. You may notice that the story has stopped again.

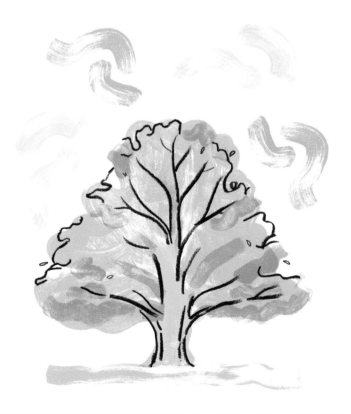

Let go of labels

Many of us have a habit of labelling ourselves and others. We say, 'She's a finance person' or 'I'm not an entrepreneur'. As you keep doing the exercises in this journal, you'll start to realize that you're far more than you've ever imagined yourself to be.

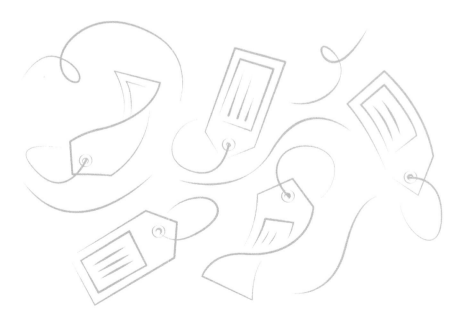

Exercise

Think back to the last time someone labelled you. How did you feel
about it? Write it down.

Someone said I wasn't very forgiving. I
felt terrible about being judged like her

Letting go of labels allows people and situations to change and develop.
Things happen more easily when we skip the labels.

Now write down all the labels you've applied to yourself:

introvert divorced intelligent not
lacking in ambition fearful caucasian ISTJ
not good at .... remembering things
good at
highly sensitive abused good mother
not a good wife good nanny good
wife old overweight self-diagnosed
lazy not a traveller home type

Exercise (continued)

Now put your pen down and look at what you've written. Using the space below, write down your answers to the following questions relating to each label you've given yourself:

- Can I be 100 per cent certain that this is true?

- Is there some pay-off from labelling myself in this way? If so, what is it?

- What's the cost of labelling myself?

- When have I lost out by doing so?

Now imagine that you've let go of these labels. How do you feel?
Write it down:

_____

_____

_____

_____

_____

_____

_____

_____

_____

_____

_____

_____

_____

_____

_____

_____

_____

_____

_____

_____

_____

_____

_____

Let go of labelling others

When we let go of labels, we see people and situations in new and different ways. Relationships improve and we create new ones. New ideas and opportunities come to us.

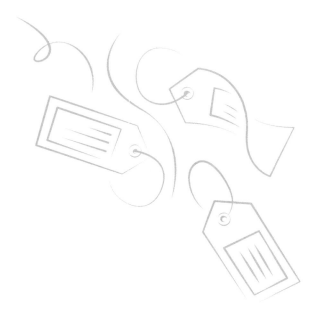

Exercise

Make a list of the people you've labelled in some way, in the space below. You can include both individuals and groups of people who share a particular nationality, race or social background. Add the labels you've attached to each of them.

_____

_____

_____

_____

_____

_____

_____

_____

_____

_____

Stop and look at what you've written. Ask yourself the following questions:

- Can I be 100 per cent certain that these labels are accurate?

- Is there some pay-off from labelling people in this way?

- How would these people feel if they found out that I'd labelled them?

- What's the cost to me of labelling these people?

- When have I lost out by doing so?

Let go of judgements

'There is nothing either good or bad, but thinking makes it so'

– William Shakespeare, *Hamlet*

Many of us have a habit of judging. We label people, events and experiences as 'good' or 'bad', but these mental labels don't exist physically. If you judge, you suffer; it's hard to do anything constructive when you're frustrated, angry or depressed. Allow judgements to come and go. If you're present you can observe judgements appearing and disappearing in your mind. You don't need to tell anyone about them. You don't need to resist them either – just watch them come and go. Once they go, something new will happen.

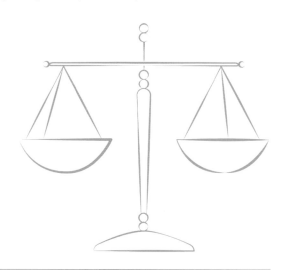

Exercise

Notice what's going on around you: the way people speak and behave, the weather, the pace at which things happen, the thoughts that appear in your mind.

If you keep returning to the present, you'll start noticing judgements as they appear: 'She shouldn't have said that', 'People shouldn't do that', 'What a stupid situation' and so on.

Instead of clinging to these judgements, just watch them come and go. Make sure you don't resist them – that only makes it harder to let go of them.

After a while the judgements will vanish. New ones may appear – you can let go of them too.

Let go of conclusions

Conclusions are closely related to stories, labels, judgements and opinions. We have a few experiences and then draw some conclusion. It could be 'Men are like this', 'Women are like that' or 'That's the way the world is'. We conclude that certain things work in certain ways.

It's OK to observe tendencies in human behaviour and the world around us, but conclusions are way more than that. The Latin root of the verb *to conclude* means *to shut completely*. When we reach a conclusion about someone or something, we shut out all other possibilities. Then we misinterpret situations and miss out on opportunities.

at everyone from a particular
haves in a certain way, you

business opportunity.
t shape our lives, and
ning. If you keep returning
e of what's going on.
isions.

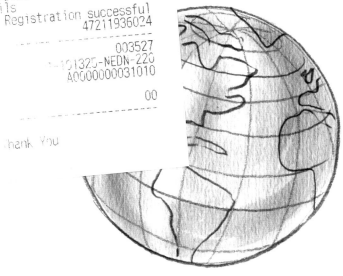

Exercise

Jot down your responses to the following and, once you've done that,
write down the events that have led you to these conclusions:

The places you don't like

[handwritten] Busy places, work places, places with people, pubs, clubs, [illegible] France, Belgium, any country, some countryside.

The kinds of people you don't like

[handwritten] loud people, chatty people, judgmental people, ex-people in my life, [illegible] people

The activities you avoid

[handwritten] everything

The situations you avoid getting into

[handwritten] confrontation - disagreements, [illegible]
[handwritten] [illegible]

Now, for each conclusion, ask yourself the following questions and write down the answers below:

- What's this conclusion costing me?

- What am I missing in life as a result of this?

- Now look at your list of conclusions again. How would you feel if you let go of them?

free

See things as they are

For several years I rented an apartment in a wealthy part of London and worked from home most of the time. When I first arrived it was common to see Porsches parked in the street. One day I was walking along when I saw a Ferrari parked on the side of the road. I stopped and looked at it more closely, and noticed that all kinds of thoughts were appearing in my mind. They weren't to do with not having a car. They were to do with money, or rather my lack of ready cash at the time. I felt frustrated and wondered if I would ever have plenty of money again.

After a while I realized I was looking at some metal painted red and some tyres made of black rubber. There was also a little yellow badge with a black horse rearing up on its hind legs – that was all.

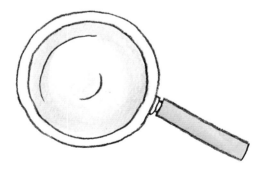

Exercise

Whenever an object catches your attention, look at it more closely.

Do you see the object for what it is, or are you lost in thoughts about something else?

Whatever the thoughts may be, keep looking. Eventually they'll die down and you'll see the object for what it is. Jot down your experience of this below:

_____

_____

_____

_____

_____

_____

_____

_____

_____

_____

_____

_____

_____

_____

Let go of shoulds

Many of us feel we should *be* this or that, or *do* this or that, or *have* this or that. When things aren't the way we think they *should* be, we judge ourselves and feel bad. We may not even realize we're doing it.

Getting your shoulds down on paper is a good start.

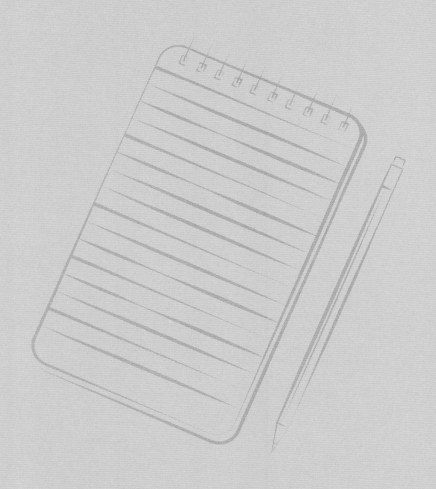

Exercise

Sit in a quiet place and make a list of all the things you feel you should be, do or have. Here are some ideas to help you get started:

- I should have done...

- I shouldn't have done...

- I should have a degree

- I should be married

- I should own my own home

- I should be wealthy by now

- I should be fitter

- I should be X kilos lighter

I should have been a better mother
I should have been a better wife/girlfriend
I should have made a success my mum
I should have a good income
I should be where I put me
I should know what I put into
I should be like as deserving

Now examine each one carefully. Where did it come from? Did someone say something that stuck in your mind? Did you pick it up from your friends, or did it come from someone in authority? Write down the answers to these questions below:

_____

_____

_____

_____

_____

_____

_____

_____

_____

_____

_____

If you examine your shoulds carefully, they'll start to lose their power over you.

Now stand up, close your eyes and shake your body – particularly your hands and feet. Shake off all the shoulds.

Now bring your attention back to the present. Notice how you feel.

It can take a while to let go of your shoulds – keep shaking them off.

Let go of expectations

'Expectation is the culprit. Let go!'

– SPH JGM Nithyananda Paramashivam

By definition, expectations aren't reality. They're just repetitive thoughts about how things should be. We get frustrated when people and situations don't meet our expectations. We keep resisting what is, and struggling against reality.

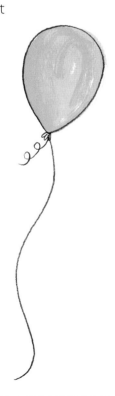

When we let go of expectations, we allow people and situations to change. If someone you're working with doesn't do what they say they will, you can point it out to them. If they still don't do it, you may need to find someone else. There's no need to get stressed about it.

Things that don't fit our expectations keep happening in the world. Some people judge what's happening, get angry, label other people and so on. In the meantime, life keeps unfolding. If we let go of our expectations and judgements, we can stay calm and take the right action at the right time. Intuition will tell you what to do (as I'll explain in the chapter *Surrender and Tune into Something Far More Intelligent than Your Brain* on page 111).

Exercise

Make a list of everything you expect to happen in your life.

_____

_____

_____

_____

_____

_____

_____

_____

Now write down how you expect people to behave. You can write down
general standards of behaviour. You can also assign specific expectations
to each person.

_____

_____

_____

_____

_____

_____

_____

_____

_____

_____

_____

This exercise may seem absurd – because it is. On the one hand there's reality, which is changing and evolving all the time. On the other hand there's the shopping list of expectations that your mind has drawn up and is now trying to impose on the world. They may be *legitimate* expectations, backed up by law or social convention, but they're still just *thoughts.* The mind is perpetually clashing with reality – guess which side is going to win.

You can tell people what you want them to do, and they may agree to do it. If they *don't* do it, you can take the appropriate action. At the same time, I recommend you *let go* of your expectations. *You're* the one who's going to suffer if you cling to them. Try this instead:

• Continue with your work and relationships in the normal way. Tell people what you want them to do. Tell them what you're going to do, and then do it. But drop your expectations.

• Be present. Observe everything that happens, moment by moment.

• Take action whenever it feels appropriate.

• How do you feel? Do you notice any difference in the way life unfolds?

Keep an open mind

If human beings were as rational as we like to think we are, we'd be open to information from any source, regardless of whether it fitted with our existing beliefs. Of course, we would check to see if the new information was accurate, but being open-minded in the first place would help us to survive and prosper. In reality, most of us suffer from *confirmation bias*: the tendency to look for information that confirms our beliefs and to ignore or fail to notice evidence that contradicts them, even if it's right in front of us.

One way to start overcoming confirmation bias is to escape from your bubble.

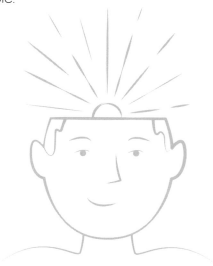

Exercise

- Buy a newspaper or visit a news website that you don't normally look at. It's best to choose one that isn't aimed at people of your social background. Experiment with seeing things from a different point of view.

- When you meet someone whose opinion is different from yours, ask them lots of questions. Let go of your opinions and listen. Learn as much as you can about what they're saying and how they see things.

- Go to a part of your city or region that you haven't visited before (provided it's safe to do so). Walk around. Watch and listen. Talk to people.

- Travel by public transport whenever possible. Put your phone away. Be present and pay attention to everything around you.

Breaking a few habits will help you to see a bigger picture. You may find yourself having new ideas and spotting new opportunities.

Practise gratitude

'You can live either in expectation or in gratitude, never in both'

– SPH JGM Nithyananda Paramashivam

Most of us have mental habits that help to keep us stuck. One of them is the habit of complaining. We can start getting rid of it by looking instead for things that make us feel grateful.

Instead of worrying about what's *going* to happen or what *has* happened, it's better to be grateful for what's *happening now*.

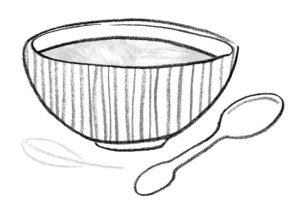

Exercise

Last thing at night, write down everything you appreciate most about today. Exclude anything that's happened before today or that might happen in the future. This exercise is purely about today. You might write about what you had for lunch or dinner, a conversation you had with a friend, the weather, something you learned, something that made you laugh, or something interesting that you saw on television or read about in the news.

Imagine giving everything away

Many of us have been taught to 'count our blessings', but we may then start to believe that what we've accumulated is 'ours'. We cling to it and become afraid of losing it.

You may be wondering what the difference is between being grateful and counting blessings. Essentially:

- Gratitude happens in the moment. You enjoy an experience and let it go.

- When you count your blessings, you label something as 'yours'. It could be a person, a physical possession, your reputation, some money...

It's better to enjoy each experience, be grateful for it and let it go.

The following exercise is from the Zen tradition:

Exercise

- When you wake up, lie still in bed for a few minutes.

- Think of your possessions and imagine yourself giving them away, one by one, starting with those you value the most.

- Once you've mentally given everything away, get up and carry on with your day as usual.

- Do this for several days in succession.

- Use the space below to write down how you feel:

Be grateful in the present moment

When we're consciously grateful once or twice a day, it spills over into the rest of our lives. We start to appreciate everything. Try this exercise:

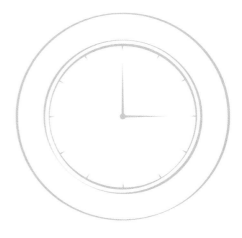

Exercise

- Notice the temperature in the room where you're sitting.

- Notice the ground beneath your feet while you're walking around.
Notice the sounds, colours and textures. Pay attention to what people
are saying as well as how they are saying it.

- Appreciate the air as it flows in and out of your body.
Notice the weather, and the temperature of the air against your skin –
and appreciate both.

- Appreciate the food you're eating, the people you're meeting, the ideas
you're sharing and the work you're doing. (If you have no work right
now, you can appreciate the opportunity to reflect, meet new people and
try new things.) Be grateful for any money you receive.

- If you're delayed, pay attention to how you feel about it.
Notice the sensations within your body, which may include tension
or irritation. Appreciate the opportunity to observe what's going on
in your mind, in your body and all around you. Be grateful for the
lessons you're learning.

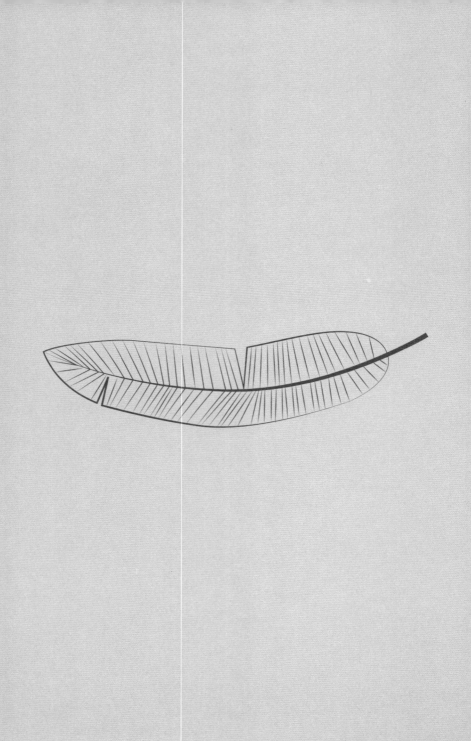

Let Go of the Pain
That Runs Your Life

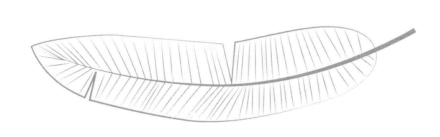

Now it's time for the second step in the three-step process:

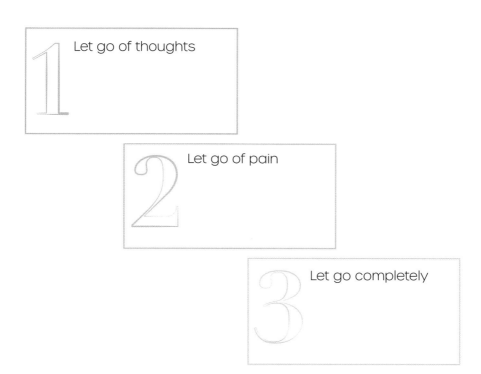

1 Let go of thoughts

2 Let go of pain

3 Let go completely

In the last chapter we practised exercises that involved observing thoughts and letting go of them. Now it's time to go deeper and consider the pain that perpetuates streams of negative thoughts.

Revisit the past

We allow pain from the past to run our lives. If you want to remove that pain, you have to take a close look at your past. This pain may be stored in your body. It's very likely that you've already had some experience of letting go of this pain. It could have been a bereavement or the end of a relationship.

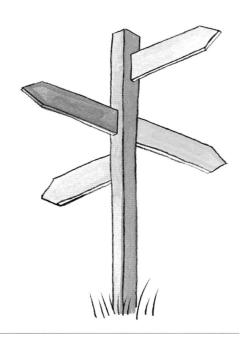

Exercise

Can you think of a time when you embraced negative emotions and gradually let go of them? Write them down below. There's no right or wrong answer, but it's nice to know your starting point.

This healing process can take a long time. Fortunately, there's a technique that is much faster and more effective (see overleaf).

Completion – re-live to relieve

I learned the Science of Completion^{SM} from SPH JGM Nithyananda Paramashivam, known to his followers as Swamiji. (The original source is the *ShivaJnana Upanishad, Vijnana Bhairava Tantra,* 94th verse, 22nd technique.)

Swamiji talks about *pain patterns,* which are mental impressions or psychological imprints. Another word for these pain patterns is *incompletions,* which he defines as 'incidents, memories and wrong cognitions from the past that are occupying our present and are affecting our future'.

Incompletions make us feel powerless. Here's an example:

A schoolteacher asks a class of five-year-old children a question. A girl raises her hand to answer it, but she gets it wrong. All her classmates laugh at her, and she feels ashamed.

Fast-forward 20 years: this 25-year-old businesswoman is doing very well in her career but is afraid of public speaking. Every time she's asked to make a presentation to an audience, she's overwhelmed by negative thoughts. 'What if I mess this up?', 'People will laugh at me' and so on. She avoids public speaking as much as possible, and her career suffers as a result. An experience at the age of five creates a pain pattern that is still running her life two decades later.

Exercise

The first and most important step is to decide that you're going to let go of the pain patterns that are holding you back. Then you make a list of the incidents that caused you pain in the past. These incidents could have occurred in any area of your life, at any time from early childhood onwards.

Use the space below to list them:

_____

_____

_____

_____

_____

_____

_____

_____

_____

_____

_____

_____

_____

_____

_____

_____

_____

Now sit in front of a mirror. Connect with yourself by looking
into your eyes. Re-live each incident intensely – at least five times –
by talking aloud to the person in the mirror. *Re-live to relieve.*
Complete with each incident over a period of 21 minutes.

Please note that you don't *recall* the incident – you *re-live* it.
If something painful happened when you were five years old, become
five years old again, with the way you saw things at that age – not the
way you see things now. The aim is to experience everything as a
five-year-old, and to allow all the feelings to come up.

(If you don't have a mirror to hand, you can simply close your eyes,
look inward and re-live the experience.)

Do this over and over again, in several sessions if you wish.

Practise completion

You can also use completion to let go of fears. Most of us are afraid of something. It could be spiders, ill health or losing our job. Some fears are rational and help us survive, but in many cases they come from negative experiences that may never be repeated. Once we identify those negative experiences we can remove the pain patterns they've created. Then we can stop worrying about the future and live our lives to the full.

How about you? What are you afraid of now, based on something that happened years ago?

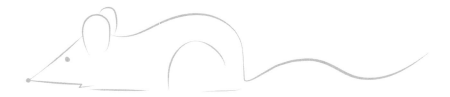

Exercise

In the space below, write down a description of everything you're afraid of. Then go back and identify the original incident that led to this fear. Use the completion exercise to re-live each experience until it loses its power over you. (This may require several sessions.)

Start discovering your inner image

We can usually trace the pain that runs our lives to a particular experience in early childhood. Imagine yourself as a tall building. Many of us present a shiny exterior to the outside world, but the inside of the building is not like that at all. Imagine that your building has an atrium containing a fast-growing weed that quickly blocks out all the light. This enormous weed is a good analogy for a pain pattern from your early childhood. It gives rise to your inner image, which is the way you see yourself.

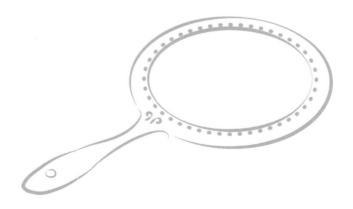

Exercise

Your inner image consists of your thoughts and feelings about yourself – the stories you tell yourself about you. Most of us aren't fully aware of what's going on. Earlier (see page 45) I asked you to write down the answers to several questions, including the following:

- What's the story you tell about yourself?

- What are the beliefs underlying your story?

Your answers to these questions will help you discover your inner image.

Sit quietly and write down below what you believe about yourself and how you feel about yourself. Write down all your thoughts and feelings – whatever comes to mind – without holding back. You're the only person who's going to see this, so write down how you really feel:

_____

_____

_____

_____

A lot of what you write may be negative and bring up strong emotions. Once we get our beliefs and feelings about ourselves down on paper, we can take a good look at them. Can you see any connection between what you've just written and what's happening in your life?

Now, turn back to the completion exercise on page 93. Identify the incident when you first came to this conclusion about yourself. Keep re-living that early, painful experience until the pain melts away.

Completion every day

The completion technique involves sitting down for a few minutes (ideally 21 minutes) at a time to re-live the experience that is causing pain, agitation or disturbance in you. Once you've done that and experienced the results, I encourage you to practise completion regularly.

The pain, suffering or discomfort will gradually dissipate, either in one session or in several sessions – depending on the intensity with which you re-live it. The more intensely you do so, the more you'll experience yourself as consciousness, which is bliss. You may also feel love, compassion, creativity – all apparently out of nowhere.

If you keep doing this, you'll start to feel lighter. The quality of your life will improve dramatically. You'll feel more and more fulfilled.

Exercise

Every time you have a painful experience, make sure you don't suppress it or try to deflect it in some way. Please do this instead:

- Turn inwards.

- Find the pain, agitation or discomfort in your body.

- Go back and find the original incident – when you first began to feel this way.

- Re-live that experience exactly as it happened, from beginning to end.

Try this throughout the day, for seven days.
Keep a list below of each time you practise completion.

_____

_____

_____

_____

_____

_____

_____

_____

_____

_____

The people you find really annoying

The problems we have with other people tend to follow a pattern – we have the same or a similar problem with different people, at different times and in different places. It could be something that happens in one job after another, one business after another or one relationship after another.

Eventually, some of us realize that we're the common factor in all these situations. We can change job, find a new partner or emigrate, but the same things keep happening.

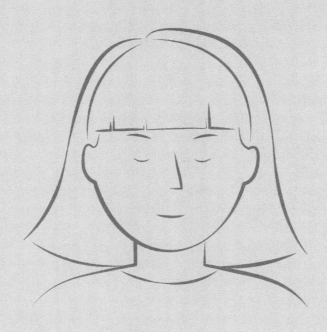

Exercise

On the left-hand side below, make a list of the people you find most annoying. Please include both individuals and types of people. They can be family, friends, colleagues and/or celebrities. Write down as many as you can – the more data you have to work with, the better.

To the right of each name on the list, write down what you find most annoying about them.

Who I find most annoying	What I find most annoying about them

Do you keep having similar problems with different people?
What are the patterns in your relationships? Write them down.

_____

_____

_____

_____

_____

_____

_____

_____

_____

_____

_____

_____

_____

_____

_____

_____

_____

_____

_____

_____

_____

Integrate your shadow and become whole

'Everything that irritates us about others can lead us to an understanding of ourselves'

– Carl Jung, *Memories, Dreams, Reflections*

You may be shocked to hear this, but the things you find annoying in other people are a reflection of *you*. The *shadow* is a term coined by Carl Jung. Another word for it is the *dark side*. It contains anything you've failed to accept about yourself, which you then project – unconsciously – onto other people. In the meantime you keep having the same problems with other people, over and over again.

The way to understand your shadow is to look at the people who annoy you most – hence the last exercise. What annoys you about them is something you've suppressed in yourself and projected onto them. Whatever it is, you'll keep seeing it in other people until you acknowledge it in yourself and embrace it.

Then you'll start to become whole.

Exercise

On pages 49–51 I asked you to write down your stories about other people – for example, people are rude, all politicians are liars, etc. Once you've identified a story you tell about others, you can turn it into a question about you. For example, 'When have I been rude?', 'When have I lied?'

Once you've identified the behaviour you've been denying in yourself, you can start to embrace it. Please note that I'm not asking you to label yourself. You're just identifying things that you're capable of being and doing. If you embrace every aspect of yourself, you'll start to become whole.

Identify your own behaviours that you have supressed, denied or simply failed to notice, and write them down below.

_____

_____

_____

_____

_____

_____

_____

_____

_____

_____

_____

Becoming whole

Trying to be good is stressful and tiring. If you decide you mustn't be judgemental, you'll find yourself constantly checking your thoughts and behaviour for any misdemeanour. You may also find yourself monitoring other people, in case they start judging anyone.

Relax. It's better to be whole than good. We can all be judgemental at times. What's the big deal? We can be anything. Let go and give yourself a break. The chaotic thoughts will continue to die down, making it much easier to be present and enjoy each moment.

It's better to accept every aspect of yourself. Accept that you can be anything.

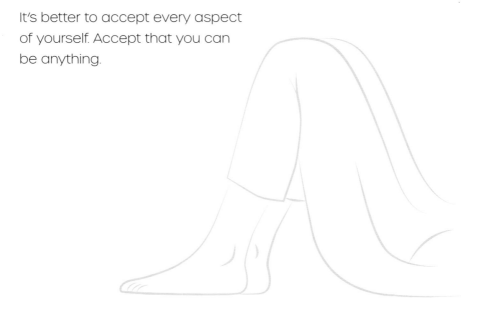

Exercise

When there's no one else around, try reading the
following statements out loud:

- I can be clever
- I can be stupid
- I can be beautiful
- I can be ugly
- I can be fat
- I can be skinny
- I can be mean
- I can be generous
- I can be kind
- I can be unkind
- I can be old
- I can be youthful
- I can be lazy
- I can be energetic
- I can be fascinating
- I can be boring
- I can be rich
- I can be poor
- I can be patient
- I can be impatient
- I can be tidy
- I can be untidy
- I can be efficient
- I can waste time

Once you realize that you can be anything, you start to become whole.
You're no longer trying to be one thing and not another. You'll feel
better about yourself – and other people will feel better around you.

Go deeper

If you've done the shadow exercises from page 102 onwards, you'll have discovered what you've been projecting onto other people. That's already a big help. You'll start to become whole.

Now we can go much deeper and experience ourselves as whole – which is our true nature – using the completion technique. We're extremely unlikely to dig out all of our incompletions in one go, but at least we're looking in the right place. The shadow exercises can help us do this. Then we can dig deeper and deeper, to get rid of all the incompletions.

Exercise

Write down the answers to the questions below. Include as much detail as possible:

What are you projecting onto other people?

_____

_____

_____

_____

_____

_____

What are the pain patterns that are causing you to do this?

_____

_____

_____

_____

_____

_____

I invite you to complete them and let them go.

Keep looking inwards. Keep digging and completing.

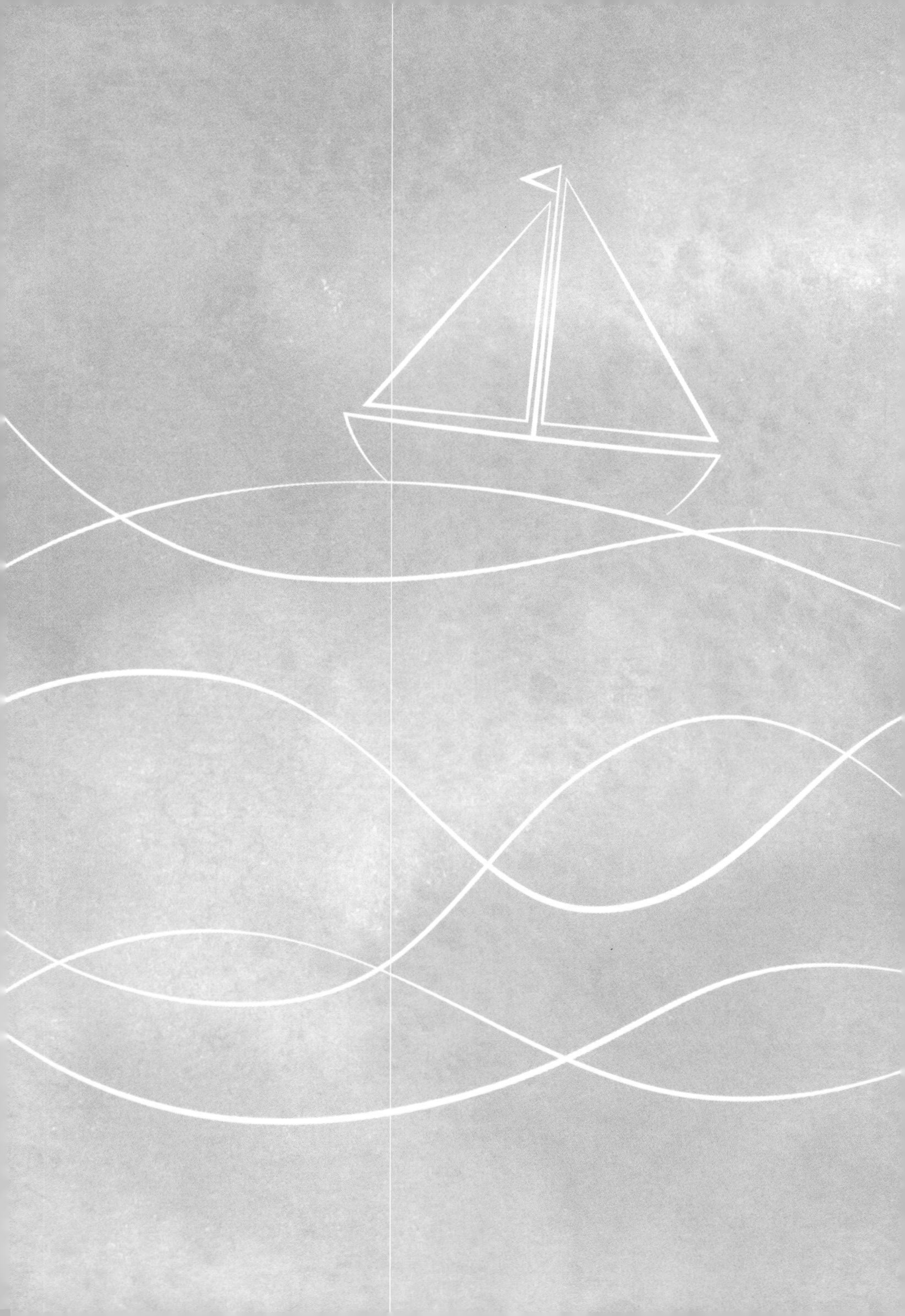

Surrender and Tune into Something Far More Intelligent than Your Brain

---

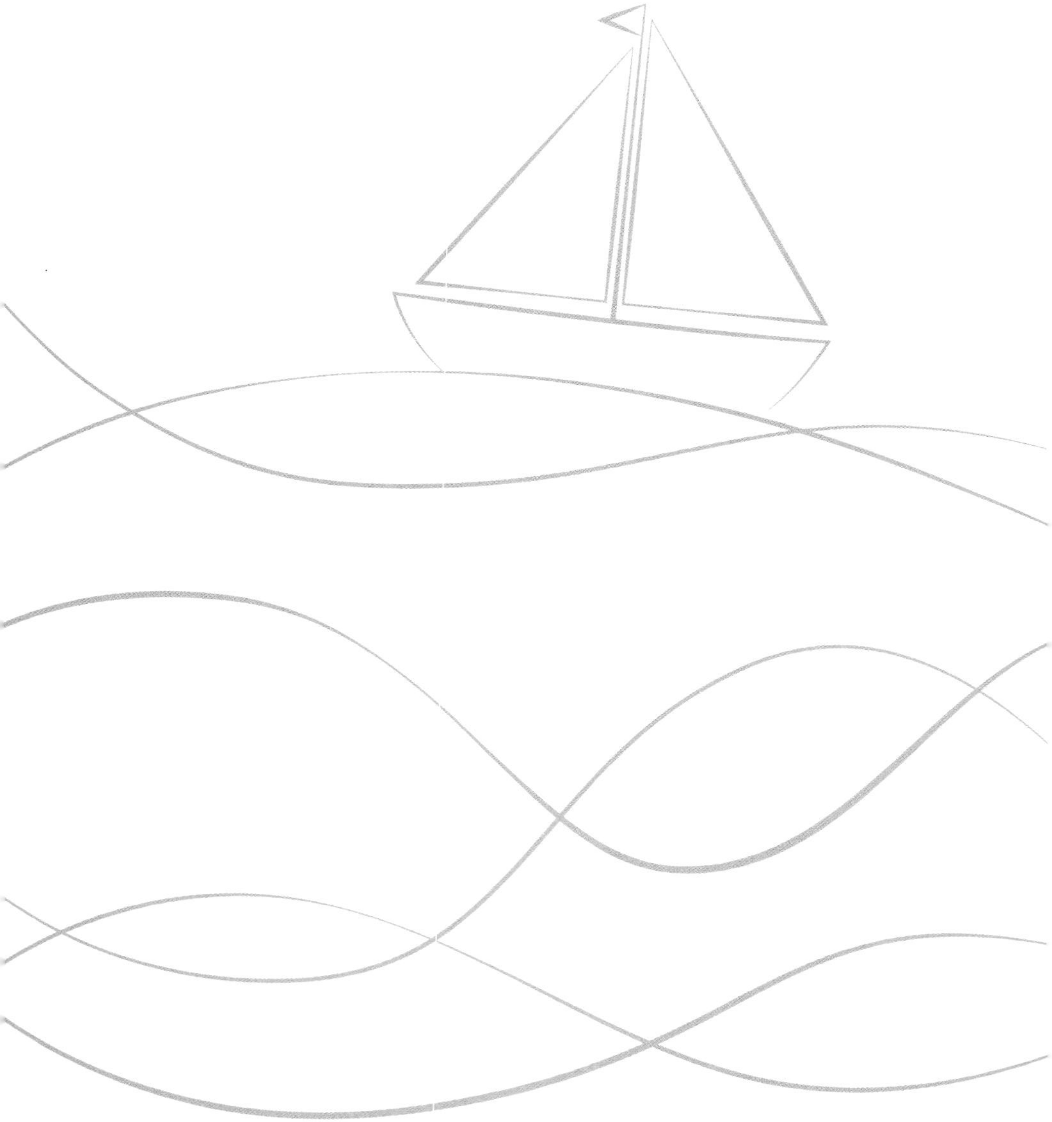

Just to recap, this is what we've covered in the first three chapters:

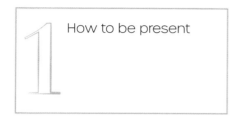
How to be present

How to let go of the thoughts that have been holding you back

How to let go of the pain that has been ruling your life

Now we've done the groundwork, we can move on to the really exciting bit, which is letting go completely. This is sometimes called surrender. I must warn you that *surrender* may seem paradoxical at first, but letting go completely is much more productive than trying to control everyone and everything. It also has the power to transform your life, so it's worth experiencing for yourself.

Apart from the first exercise, this chapter will consist of insights (see pages 118–30). I invite you to contemplate each insight and write down your thoughts in the space on the right-hand side.

How to surrender

If you've done the exercises earlier in the book you'll have started letting go of negative thoughts and emotions. Now it's time to let go completely.

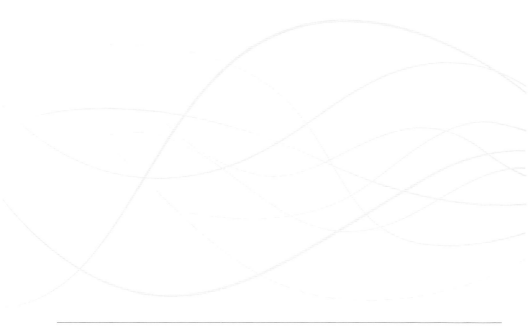

Exercise

Forget about the past and the future. Forget about your goals, plans and expectations. Let go of all your memories. Drop all your thoughts about the present, including judgements, labels and expectations. Close your eyes and imagine yourself throwing them all away.

Now do whatever feels appropriate, moment by moment. If you keep a to-do list, pick the item that needs your attention now and work on it.

Follow your intuition – do whatever feels right, moment by moment*.

Let go of any thoughts about the outcome. Don't bother thinking about results. Just immerse yourself in whatever you're doing and enjoy it.

*Don't mistake incompletions for intuition. If you're present you can observe thoughts as they arise, as I described earlier (see page 24). However, the question is, are those thoughts coming from your intuition or from incompletions? Some people think they're using their intuition when they're really acting out of fear and incompletion. They're being triggered by unconscious pain patterns that haven't been completed. The way to avoid this is to make sure you keep completing the pain that is stored in your system. Intuition is based on love, not fear.

Pure consciousness

Remember the thoughts that keep you stuck, from earlier in the book? All that stuff about not being good enough, being a winner, being a loser? The exercises you've done since then will help you let go of the stories that have been holding you back.

Now for another weird bit. When you surrender, you let go of both the stories *and* the person who appears in them. S/he is just a story too. When we're born we simply are. As small babies we have experiences, we laugh and we cry, but we don't yet have a story about ourselves as a person. That comes later. By the time you're an adult, you've accumulated lots of episodes describing what you see as 'your' adventures, achievements, suffering and so on.

So, what's the alternative? What if you aren't the person in the story? Who are you? The answer is that you simply are. You're consciousness. Thoughts, emotions and sensations appear and disappear within consciousness. It's like a film being projected onto a screen. You're the screen, not the film.

Once we realize that we are consciousness – and let go completely – it gives a tremendous feeling of space, in which there are infinite possibilities.

Exercise

Let's consider a couple of examples of pure consciousness:

• You wake up naturally, without an alarm. For at least a moment or two, there are no thoughts. Gradually, you begin to notice your surroundings. You wonder what time it is, and you think about breakfast. The thoughts have started up again, and may continue for the rest of the day.

• You're standing on top of a mountain – or on a clifftop – in front of a scene so beautiful that your mind falls still. Maybe the stillness lasts for only a few moments. Then the thoughts start up again: 'Should I take a photo?, 'Who's that person over there?'

• Write down a time when you were conscious without any thoughts – perhaps only for a few seconds.

_____

_____

_____

_____

_____

_____

_____

_____

_____

_____

_____

Insight 1: Once you surrender, your inner image will bother you less

1 In the last chapter, I talked about your inner image (or self-image) as opposed to your outer image, which you project to others, as though you're wearing a mask.

The gap between the inner image and the outer image causes all kinds of problems. As Swamiji points out, when we complete and surrender, our low inner image becomes inactive. It's there as a piece of historical information that we may think about from time to time but that no longer causes us pain or runs our life.

For example, when I complete and surrender, I let go of my identity as John Purkiss and just flow. One thing happens after another, with no worries about what's going to happen to John Purkiss, what other people think about John Purkiss, etc. It's far more enjoyable than the old, restricted way of living.

I encourage you to surrender and experience this for yourself.

Exercise

Consider this lesson and let go completely. Your intuition will tell you
what to do. Jot down your thoughts in the space below.

Insight 2: Surrender will change the way you see yourself and the world

2

We try to get what we want, in the hope that we'll be happy when we do so, at some point in the future. Eventually we discover that it doesn't work. Fortunately, there's an alternative – surrender.

When we let go completely, things fall into place. Surrender isn't giving up or doing nothing. It just means that we stop trying to make the world conform to our fixed ideas about how things should be. When we surrender we create space for something more exciting to happen. This raises a question: What's the 'something else' that makes everything happen?

The answer is beyond time and space. It's beyond name and form. One word we can use to describe it is 'Existence', by which I mean the intelligence that is running everything, including your brain, your body and everything around you, such as plants, animals, humans, planets and stars. It's easier to surrender once we realize that we're part of Existence and it's constantly supporting us.

Exercise

Write down one or more examples of when Existence has supported you.
You didn't know how things would work out, but they did.

_____

_____

_____

_____

_____

_____

_____

_____

_____

_____

_____

_____

_____

_____

_____

_____

_____

_____

_____

_____

Insight 3: The ego is the illusion that you're separate from Existence

3

You aren't the body or the mind. These come and go. You're pure consciousness, which witnesses the body changing and the thoughts coming and going. You have a choice: You can either try to achieve everything through physical and mental effort; or surrender and follow your intuition, only thinking and taking action when necessary. For many, the first option works well for a time, but eventually it stops working and we run into a wall.

Eventually, some of us realize that it isn't a wall – it's a big step. If we want to keep moving forwards, we have to go up a level. And we need to let go of something before we can do that. Once we work out what we need to let go of, we move up and keep moving forwards for a while, until we hit another wall. This process is all about letting go. We let go of judgements, labels, painful memories, mental patterns, preconceptions and so on. The higher we go, the further we can see. We feel lighter and things happen more easily.

Exercise

Consider this insight. When has trying to achieve everything through physical and mental effort stopped working for you? Use the space below to write down your answers.

_____

_____

_____

_____

_____

_____

_____

_____

_____

_____

_____

_____

_____

_____

_____

_____

_____

_____

_____

Insight 4: Once you surrender, your intuition will tell you what to do

Once you surrender, you can relax and enjoy the process. Your mind will become quieter because you're no longer resisting what's happening now, harking back to the past or fantasizing about the future. Then your intuition will tell you what to do.

Some people worry that they'll become disorganized if they surrender. However, there's no conflict between surrender and organizing things in your professional and personal life. If you surrender, your intuition will tell you when it is and isn't necessary. You'll organize things faster when your mind is clear.

Exercise

How has your intuition helped you in the past? Write it down:

_____

_____

_____

_____

_____

_____

_____

_____

_____

_____

_____

_____

_____

_____

_____

_____

_____

_____

_____

_____

_____

_____

Insight 5: Surrender during conversations

Some people try to control conversations, to impose their point of view. It's better to let go and listen with an open mind. While you're listening, you'll notice thoughts and feelings that come up in reaction to what other people are saying. It's best to observe this mental chatter and let it go.

If you surrender during conversations, you may notice some remarkable changes. You'll get on better with whoever you're listening to. Eventually, you may find yourself listening in what feels like an empty space. There are no separate people – only sounds and images, and then thoughts and feelings, that appear and disappear. You just notice whatever comes up and let it go. You learn a lot. New ideas appear during the conversation. They can come from either person – it doesn't matter who.

It's best to be empty and listen. Allow the other person to talk. When they've finished speaking, it may or may not occur to you to say something. Sometimes the best response is silence. Sometimes it's best to ask a question, so you can understand what they're saying in more detail. All you have to do is let go and be present.

Exercise

Next time you have a conversation with someone, try allowing yourself
to be empty and listen. Write down your experiences below:

_____

_____

_____

_____

_____

_____

_____

_____

_____

_____

_____

_____

_____

_____

_____

_____

_____

_____

_____

_____

_____

_____

Insight 6: If you're present and let go, there will be helpful coincidences

6

Many of us have noticed periods in our lives when everything seemed to flow naturally, without any major obstacles. If you're present and you let go, this may happen frequently. People appear at just the right time. Circumstances change. Things fall into place. It can feel uncanny and send a shiver down your spine.

You may have heard people say, 'There's no such thing as coincidence'. This is based on a linguistic misunderstanding.

Coincidence just means that two things happen at the same time. It doesn't mean it's random or accidental. At the deepest level there's no separation: cause and effect are one. Things unfold, sometimes in ways that the mind struggles to comprehend or explain. But we don't need to worry about the mind. We can just let go.

Exercise

Think of any times in your life when you've experienced helpful
coincidences. Write them down:

_____

_____

_____

_____

_____

_____

_____

_____

_____

_____

_____

_____

_____

_____

_____

_____

_____

_____

_____

_____

_____

Insight 7: Embrace uncertainty

7

Many of us are afraid of uncertainty – a lot of investors are. Whenever there's a crisis, people sell their investments in a hurry. Even when there isn't a crisis, many of us try to remove uncertainty from our lives in the hope of feeling 'safe' one day.

The certainty we're pursuing is a mirage: life is uncertain. As you practise the exercises in this journal, you'll become more comfortable with uncertainty. In the beginning you may see yourself as a separate body/mind trying to make your way through life. The more you let go of the thoughts and feelings that have been holding you back, the more you'll realize that you *aren't* separate. Keep surrendering and everything will flow.

Exercise

Think of any times in your life when you accepted that you didn't know
what was going to happen – then something wonderful happened.
Write them down:

_____

_____

_____

_____

_____

_____

_____

_____

_____

_____

_____

_____

_____

_____

_____

_____

_____

_____

_____

_____

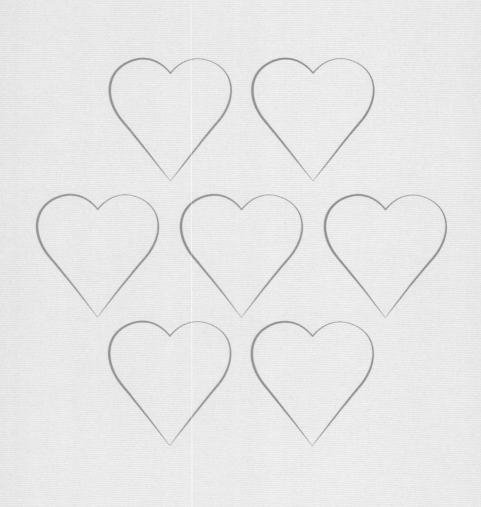

Turn Your Desires into Reality by Letting Go

So far I've talked about how to:

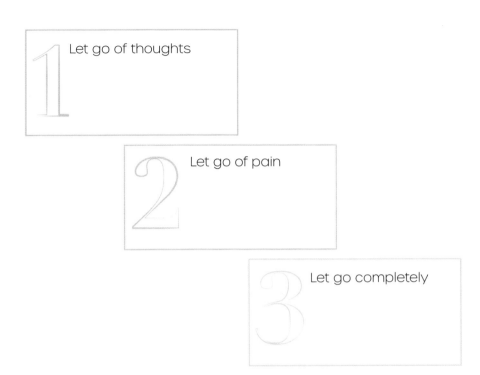

1   Let go of thoughts

2   Let go of pain

3   Let go completely

Now it's time to come back to the question I asked you right at the beginning: 'What do you want to change in your life?' In other words, which desires do you want to turn into reality?

We manifest our *beliefs*, not our *desires*. Once you're complete, your beliefs and desires become one. Then your desires start to become reality.

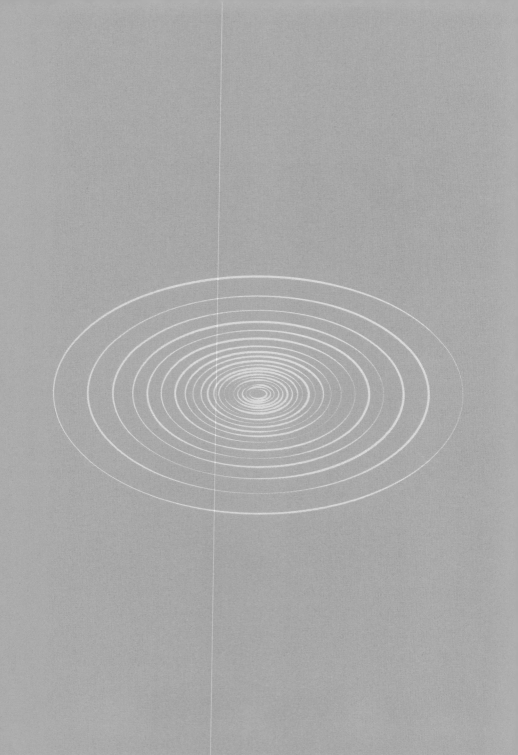

Where do desires come from?

We can divide desires into three categories:

1. Desires that come from the ego

The ego is made up of incompletions, which I described earlier. When we're incomplete, we pursue desires based on fear and greed, which leads to more incompletion and suffering. One example is eating as much food as possible, out of an unconscious fear that there won't be enough food in the near future. Completion will help you to remove these desires.

2. Borrowed desires

These are desires that we've 'borrowed' from other people. For example, it could be a desire to have a big car because your best friend wants a big car.

3. Desires that arise naturally

Once we remove ego-based desires and borrowed desires, we're left with desires that arise naturally. These desires simply occur in us.

What's stopping your desires from becoming reality?

If your inner space is pure consciousness, natural desires are realized easily. However, in most cases, our inner space contains lots of incompletions, which are to do with what we don't want. We've come to the wrong conclusions about ourselves, other people and the world around us. When this happens, we manifest our negative beliefs instead of manifesting our natural desires.

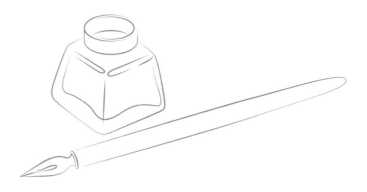

If you look carefully at your life, you can see what's happening. As I mentioned in the introduction, most of us are worried or feel stuck in one or more areas of our lives. So we keep struggling with the same issues, whether it's ill health, poor relationships, career frustrations or lack of money. None of these are random processes. These patterns of 'stuckness' repeat themselves in a way that is particular to each of us, because we each have our own particular incompletions.

One of the most popular free courses run by Swamiji's *sangha* (community) is Kalpataru™ – named after a wish-fulfilling tree in Hindu scriptures. The course includes an exercise in which you write down *one thing* that you want to happen in your life, which hasn't happened yet.

Writing down what you want to happen will show you what's stopping it from happening, so try the exercise on the next page.

Exercise

First, sit quietly on your own, with no mobile phone or other distractions. In the space below, write down something that you really want to happen in your life:

_____

_____

_____

_____

_____

_____

_____

_____

Now sit in silence and listen carefully. Your mind will start telling you why it can't happen. Please write it all down:

_____

_____

_____

_____

_____

_____

_____

_____

All these reasons why your desires can't happen are incompletions/pain patterns. Now look at each incompletion you've written down – one at a time. Do the completion exercise (see page 93) with each of them.

Identify the incident when each pain pattern started. What happened? Write it down:

_____

_____

_____

_____

_____

_____

_____

_____

_____

_____

_____

_____

_____

_____

Re-live each incident – at least five times – by talking to the person in the mirror. Allow everything that makes you powerless to come to the surface and leave your system. Feel it intensely and let it go. The decision to complete is more than 80 per cent of the battle. Once we decide to complete, it begins to happen.

Build completion into your daily routine

It's best to set aside time and do regular completion sessions. This is spiritual work. It's the equivalent of push-ups, swimming or walking up flights of stairs. If you do it regularly, your life will change. I often complete last thing at night, before I go to bed. I sleep a lot better as a result. First thing in the morning is also a great time to do completion. This is how you'll be able to tell that completion is starting to work for you:

- It becomes harder to remember the thing(s) that used to cause you so much pain.

- You no longer feel powerless when you come into contact with other people.

- You feel lighter and/or happier, for no apparent reason.

- Things start changing and happening in your life.

On page 98, I encouraged you to practise completion throughout the day. Now I recommend you build it into your routine by completing every morning and/or evening.

Exercise

• For the next seven days, practise completion first thing in the morning or last thing at night. If you're still doing the gratitude exercise (see page 79), it's best to do the completion exercise beforehand.

• First you use completion to remove the pain patterns. Then you write down what you're grateful for. You'll feel better afterwards.

• Use the space below to make notes on your completion and gratitude exercises over the course of the next seven days:

_____

_____

_____

_____

_____

_____

_____

_____

_____

_____

_____

_____

_____

_____

Notice what happens when you complete

Believe it or not, completion can be fun. It's a bit like clearing out your apartment to make space for nice, new furniture. You get rid of painful memories and out-of-date thought patterns, so something new and exciting can happen.

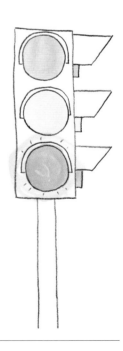

Exercise

- Re-live the experience from beginning to end. Feel any pain, irritation or discomfort that comes up.

- Notice when things suddenly open up and start happening, when you weren't really thinking about what you wanted to happen.

- Make a note to remind yourself below:

_____

_____

_____

_____

_____

_____

_____

_____

_____

_____

_____

_____

_____

_____

_____

_____

_____

Letting go allows our desires to be realized in the best possible way

Before I discovered the techniques I've explained in this book, I spent years doing the following. Maybe you've had a similar experience:

1. You set a goal;

2. You formulate an action plan;

3. You take lots of action;

4. You try to get other people to do what you want them to do (which annoys some of them);

5. If the plan doesn't work, you formulate a new plan and start again.

It's demoralizing and exhausting. Years can go by and you're no further forward. These days my approach is completely different.

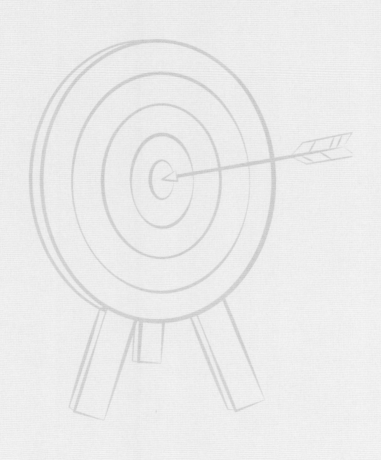

Exercise

Think about an idea you want to turn into reality. Then do this:

1. Write your idea down below:

_____

_____

_____

_____

_____

_____

_____

_____

2. Close your eyes, turn inwards, and listen to your mind telling you all the reasons why it can't happen. Write it all down:

_____

_____

_____

_____

_____

_____

_____

_____

_____

3. Go back and identify the painful experiences that you haven't completed – which are generating all the pain, discomfort, agitation and resistance.

4. Complete these experiences. Re-live to relieve.

5. Surrender and follow your intuition. It will tell you what to do.

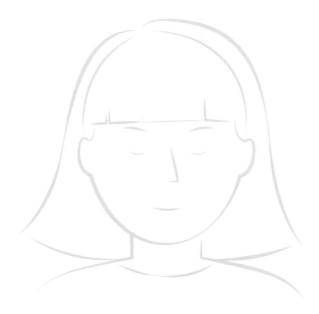

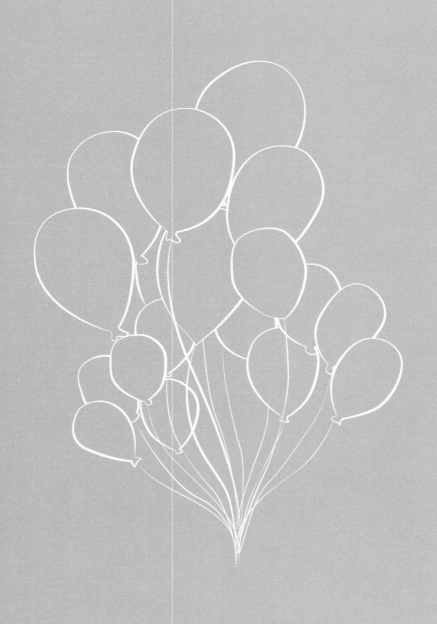

Conclusion

Most of us want to change something in our lives. Instead of working harder and harder, you can change your life much more easily by letting go. Then you'll follow your intuition and take the right action at the right time. Increasingly, you'll find yourself in the right place at the right time too.

The starting point for letting go is to be present – to keep bringing our attention back to the present moment.

Once we've learned to be present, we can take the first step. We start observing our thoughts and letting go of them. There are stories, labels, judgements, expectations, comparisons, conclusions and so on. Most are useless. Some are potentially harmful. The important thing is not to identify with them. They aren't you.

The second step is to let go of the pain that runs our lives. This requires us to look deep inside ourselves. We've all had painful experiences – many of them during early childhood – that continue to mess up our lives, years or even decades later. Unfortunately, we've suppressed these negative emotions. We may think or say we're fine, but we aren't living the lives we want. The solution is to go back and find the incident at the source of this pain pattern. Something happened that led you to draw incorrect conclusions about yourself, other people and/or the world. That pain pattern is still running your life. It makes you powerless. Now it's time to connect with yourself by looking in the mirror and re-living the painful experience. Re-live to relieve.

Once you've completed each experience, the pain pattern will lose its grip on you and your life will change for the better.

The third step is to let go completely – otherwise known as surrender. When we surrender we fall into the present. What a relief. We stop identifying with the body/mind known as John Purkiss, Frida Smith or whoever. We become one with Existence. Everything flows. We don't need to worry about the past or the future. We follow our intuition and everything falls into place – often in unexpected ways.

Once you've let go completely, your desires will become reality much more easily than before. Whatever you hold in your inner space is what you create outside. If action is required, it's quick and efficient. Things start happening, sometimes very fast indeed.

This is a journey towards consciousness. We become conscious of the thoughts and the pain patterns that are holding us back – and we let go of them. When we let go completely, we realize we're consciousness itself.

Wishing you bliss and fulfilment.

JP 😊

A Note from the Author

In 2014 I was introduced to The Supreme Pontiff of Hinduism, Jagatguru Mahasannidhanam, His Divine Holiness Bhagavan Sri Nithyananda Paramashivam (Swamiji) whom I've mentioned several times in this book. He's reviving the entire Vedic tradition from its original sources and making it accessible to everyone.

From Swamiji I learned the Science of Completion^{SM} described on page 93. If you type 'Nithyananda' and 'completion' into the search box on YouTube, you'll find many videos on this subject. I've found Swamiji's completion technique highly effective in removing the pain patterns from which the ego is constructed. The more I let go of them, the more I experience pure consciousness and bliss.

Swamiji and his *sangha* (community) run a wide range of programmes, many of which are free of charge. They include the completion technique and how to turn your desires into reality.

These teachings are available to everyone. All we need to do is let go of any preconceptions that are holding us back. I encourage you to do so.

Further information is available from www.kailaasa.org

Notes

Picture Credits

Line illustrations by Ella McLean.

Additional credits: 3 rawpixel; 8, 110 backgrounds by ninamaina/Shutterstock; 81 Yderbisheva/Dreamstime.com; 159 photo Laurence Taylor.

About the Author

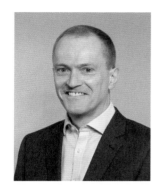

John Purkiss studied economics at the University of Cambridge and has an MBA (Master of Business Administration) from INSEAD. He began his career in banking and management consultancy, in London and Chicago, and worked in sales and marketing in the UK and continental Europe. John then learned to meditate, which made his intuition much stronger and enabled him to move into executive search. He recruits senior executives and board members, and also invests in high-growth companies.

www.johnpurkiss.com

The exercises and insights in this journal are taken from John Purkiss's original bestselling book, *The Power of Letting Go.*

John Purkiss

The Power of Letting Go

How to drop everything that's
holding you back

You're welcome to join the discussion on Facebook at:

www.facebook.com/groups/thepoweroflettinggo